The Ultimate Tylenol 8 Hour Arthritis Pain Tablets (Acetaminophen) User Guide

Safe Usage, Benefits, Dosage Guidelines, and Precautions for Effective Relief

Dr. Dorian Kevelle

Table of Contents

Introduction

Understanding Arthritis Pain and Treatment Options

Arthritis is a condition that affects the joints, causing stiffness, swelling, and pain that can make everyday tasks feel difficult. The pain often comes from inflammation inside the joints, where the protective cartilage wears down or becomes irritated. Over time, this discomfort can interfere with walking, climbing stairs, or even holding objects. There are many types of arthritis, but the most common are osteoarthritis and rheumatoid arthritis. Each has different causes, but both bring ongoing joint pain that can affect quality of life.

When it comes to treatment, doctors usually recommend a mix of approaches rather than one single method. Lifestyle changes such as regular exercise, gentle stretching, and maintaining a healthy weight are often encouraged because they ease pressure on the joints. Physical therapy can also help improve flexibility and strength. For many people, medication becomes a key part of treatment. Over-the-counter pain relievers, prescription drugs, and even injections may be used depending on how severe the pain is. Some cases may even require surgery. Still, for many individuals, pain-relieving medicines like acetaminophen are often the first choice because they can reduce discomfort without some of the stomach issues linked to other options.

Why Tylenol 8 Hour is Commonly Recommended

Tylenol 8 Hour Arthritis Pain Tablets are often recommended because they provide steady relief for long periods of time. Unlike regular pain relievers that may wear off in a few hours, this medicine is designed to work slowly in the body, offering up to eight hours of comfort. This makes it easier for people to go through their day without needing to take multiple doses. For someone living with arthritis, that can mean getting through work, enjoying time with family, or even sleeping better at night.

Another reason Tylenol is commonly recommended is because it does not contain ingredients like ibuprofen or aspirin, which can irritate the stomach or increase the risk of bleeding. This makes it a safer option for people who cannot take nonsteroidal anti-inflammatory drugs (NSAIDs). Acetaminophen, the active ingredient in Tylenol, works differently. It focuses mainly on reducing pain and lowering fever, but it does not directly reduce inflammation. Even so, for many arthritis sufferers, less pain means better movement and more freedom in daily life. Doctors often trust Tylenol as a first step because it has a long history of safe use when taken properly and is available without a prescription.

Purpose of This Guide

The purpose of this guide is to give clear and helpful information to anyone considering or already using Tylenol 8 Hour Arthritis Pain Tablets. Many people rely on pain relief medications but may not fully understand how to use them safely or what to expect. This guide is meant to take away confusion by breaking things down in plain, simple language. You will find details on how the medicine works, how to take it properly, and what risks to be aware of.

It also aims to help you make better choices by comparing Tylenol with other treatment options. Sometimes, a small change in how or when you take the medicine can make a big difference in comfort. Beyond that, the guide will also talk about lifestyle habits, precautions, and ways to use Tylenol as part of a bigger plan to manage arthritis pain. The goal is not just to explain the product, but also to support you in living a more active, less painful life. By the end, you should feel more confident about using this medication safely and making it work for your personal needs.

Chapter 1: Understanding Tylenol 8 Hour Arthritis Pain Tablets

What Acetaminophen Does in the Body

Acetaminophen, the main ingredient in Tylenol 8 Hour Arthritis Pain Tablets, works differently from many other pain relievers. Instead of directly reducing swelling like some medications do, it focuses on changing the way the brain and nervous system sense pain. When you take acetaminophen, it is absorbed into the bloodstream and travels to the brain. There, it blocks certain chemicals called prostaglandins, which normally send signals of pain and discomfort. By lowering the effect of these chemicals, acetaminophen reduces the intensity of pain that you feel.

Another important role of acetaminophen is lowering fever. It acts on the part of the brain that controls body temperature, helping bring down a fever safely. However, it does not reduce inflammation in the joints or tissues, which is why it is often recommended for pain rather than swelling. Because of its unique action, acetaminophen is considered gentle on the stomach compared to some other medicines. It doesn't usually cause irritation or bleeding in the stomach lining, making it a common choice for long-term conditions like arthritis. In simple terms, acetaminophen works by calming pain signals and helping the body feel more comfortable without heavily affecting other organs.

Key Features and Benefits of the 8 Hour Formula

The Tylenol 8 Hour Arthritis Pain Tablets are designed with a special extended-release formula that makes them different from regular acetaminophen tablets. Instead of wearing off quickly, these tablets are made to release medicine gradually over time. This allows for long-lasting relief—up to eight hours—without needing to take a pill every few hours. For someone living with arthritis, where pain can persist all day, this steady relief can make daily life much easier.

Another important feature is convenience. Fewer doses mean fewer chances of forgetting or missing a pill. This helps people stay consistent with their pain management and reduces the stress of frequent dosing schedules. The tablets are also easy to swallow, and because acetaminophen is gentle on the stomach, they can usually be taken without food.

The benefits go beyond just easing arthritis pain. The extended formula helps maintain a more even level of comfort throughout the day, making activities like walking, cooking, or working less difficult. Since acetaminophen does not generally cause drowsiness, people can take these tablets and still go about their daily responsibilities. Overall, the 8 Hour formula combines long-lasting relief, ease of use, and stomach safety, making it a trusted option for many people managing chronic pain.

How It Differs from Other Pain Relievers

Tylenol 8 Hour Arthritis Pain Tablets stand out because they contain acetaminophen, which works differently than nonsteroidal anti-inflammatory drugs (NSAIDs) like ibuprofen or naproxen. NSAIDs reduce pain by fighting inflammation in the joints and tissues, which is helpful for swelling. However, they can irritate the stomach, raise blood pressure, or even affect the kidneys when used for long periods. Acetaminophen, on the other hand, does not target inflammation but focuses on easing the way the brain interprets pain signals. This makes it a safer option for people who cannot tolerate NSAIDs or who have medical conditions that make NSAID use risky.

Another difference is in side effects. Acetaminophen is much less likely to cause stomach ulcers, heart problems, or bleeding, which are potential issues with long-term NSAID use. This is why doctors often recommend it for older adults or those with sensitive stomachs. However, acetaminophen must be taken carefully to avoid liver damage, especially when combined with alcohol or taken in higher-than-recommended doses.

In summary, while NSAIDs and acetaminophen both relieve pain, they do so in very different ways. Acetaminophen is often preferred for its stomach-friendly profile and safe long-term use, especially for people managing ongoing conditions like arthritis.

Chapter 2: Safe and Effective Usage

Recommended Dosage for Adults and Seniors

For adults and seniors, the usual recommended dose of Tylenol 8 Hour Arthritis Pain Tablets is **two caplets every 8 hours as needed**. Each caplet contains 650 mg of acetaminophen, so the maximum in a single dose is 1,300 mg. The most important rule to remember is that you should not take more than **six caplets in a 24-hour period**. This equals 3,900 mg of acetaminophen, which is the safe daily limit for this specific product. Going above this limit can cause serious liver damage, even if you feel fine in the moment. Seniors should be especially careful, as the body processes medications more slowly with age. If you have liver problems, consume alcohol regularly, or are taking other medicines that may contain acetaminophen, speak with your doctor before using it. The tablets are designed to give steady relief, so you don't need to take them too often. Following the dosage instructions strictly is the best way to get effective pain relief while staying safe.

Timing and Duration of Relief

Tylenol 8 Hour Arthritis Pain Tablets are made with an extended-release formula, meaning they work slowly over time. After taking a dose, the medication starts working within about **30 to 45 minutes**, although the exact timing may vary from person to person. Once it begins working, the relief can last up to **eight hours**, which is why it is often recommended for people dealing with ongoing arthritis discomfort throughout the day. Unlike some pain relievers that wear off quickly, this formula is designed to keep a steady amount of acetaminophen in your system, so the pain relief doesn't suddenly disappear. Because of the long duration, it's important not to take another dose too soon. Doing so could lead to accidental overdose, even if the pain feels strong. To make the most of its effects, try to take it at regular intervals that match your daily routine—such as in the morning, afternoon, and before bed—without exceeding the daily maximum. The timing gives you continuous relief, helping you stay active and comfortable without constantly worrying about when to take your next pill.

When and How to Take the Tablets

Tylenol 8 Hour Arthritis Pain Tablets are easy to take, but using them the right way makes a big difference. The tablets should be swallowed whole with a full glass of water. **Do not crush, break, or chew them.** Because they are extended-release, damaging the tablet can cause all the medicine to be released at once, which is unsafe. You can take them with or without food, but if you have a sensitive stomach, taking them after a meal may be more comfortable. It's also important to pay attention to other medications you are taking. Many over-the-counter cold, flu, or pain products contain acetaminophen. Accidentally combining them with Tylenol 8 Hour could push you past the safe daily limit. A simple way to stay safe is to keep a written record of when you take each dose. If you forget a dose, wait until it's time for the next one instead of doubling up. For people with ongoing arthritis pain, some find it helpful to plan doses around daily activities, such as before exercise or bedtime. Taking the tablets in a consistent and careful way ensures maximum relief while protecting your health.

Chapter 3: Safety Guidelines and Precautions

Important Warnings and Risk Factors

Tylenol 8 Hour Arthritis Pain Tablets can be very helpful, but like any medicine, they come with warnings you need to take seriously. The biggest risk with acetaminophen is **liver damage**. Taking more than the recommended dose, or mixing it with alcohol, greatly increases this danger. Even healthy people can harm their liver if they take too much at once or spread out too many doses in a day.

Another risk factor is **long-term use**. While this medication is designed for extended pain relief, using it daily for long periods without medical supervision may hide other health issues or put extra stress on your liver.

People with pre-existing liver disease, heavy drinkers, or those who take other medications containing acetaminophen are at higher risk. Overdose is not always obvious right away—symptoms like nausea, fatigue, or stomach pain may appear late, making it even more important to follow directions closely.

Always check the labels of cold, flu, or other pain medicines you might be using, because many already contain acetaminophen. Combining them without realizing it could push you above the safe daily limit. Following the dosage guide and staying alert to risks is the best way to stay safe.

Who Should Avoid or Limit Use

Not everyone should use Tylenol 8 Hour Arthritis Pain Tablets the same way. Some people need to avoid it completely, while others should only take it with caution and under a doctor's supervision.

People with liver problems—such as hepatitis, cirrhosis, or past liver injuries—should usually avoid this medicine because their body cannot process it safely. **Heavy alcohol users** are also at risk, since alcohol and acetaminophen together increase the chance of severe liver damage.

Children under 12 years old should not take this specific product, as it is made for adults and seniors with arthritis pain. If a child needs pain relief, there are different forms and doses designed for them.

Pregnant or breastfeeding women should check with their doctor before using it. While acetaminophen is generally considered safe in pregnancy, long-term or high-dose use should only happen under medical advice.

People with **kidney disease, malnutrition, or certain chronic illnesses** may also need to limit use, since their body might have trouble breaking down the medicine. If you're unsure whether this medication is right for you, it's always best to ask a healthcare provider before starting.

Possible Drug Interactions

Tylenol 8 Hour Arthritis Pain Tablets may seem simple, but they can interact with other medicines in ways that cause harm. The most important thing to know is that **any product**

containing acetaminophen should be avoided at the same time. Many cold, flu, and pain remedies already include it, and combining them can lead to an overdose without realizing it.

Alcohol is another major interaction. Drinking while taking acetaminophen raises the risk of liver damage. Even moderate alcohol use can be unsafe when combined with regular doses of Tylenol.

Certain **prescription drugs** may also interact. For example, some seizure medications, like carbamazepine or phenytoin, and tuberculosis medicines, such as isoniazid, can put extra stress on the liver when used with acetaminophen. People who take blood thinners like **warfarin** should also be careful, since regular use of Tylenol can affect how the blood clots and may raise the risk of bleeding.

Even natural remedies and herbal supplements can play a role. Some may increase liver stress or change how the body processes the drug. That's why it's always wise to let your doctor or pharmacist know about every medication, supplement, or vitamin you take before using Tylenol 8 Hour Arthritis Pain Tablets.

Chapter 4: Side Effects and What to Expect

Common Mild Reactions

Like most medicines, Tylenol 8 Hour Arthritis Pain Tablets (acetaminophen) can cause some mild reactions. These are usually not dangerous, and many people may not experience them at all. However, it's good to know what to expect. Some of the most common mild effects include slight nausea, upset stomach, or a feeling of discomfort after taking the tablets. Others might notice a mild headache, tiredness, or a small change in appetite. Occasionally, people report feeling dizzy or experiencing mild itching. These effects are often temporary and may go away on their own as your body adjusts to the medicine. Drinking water, taking the tablets with a light meal, and following the correct dosage can help reduce these mild issues. The key thing to remember is that these reactions are generally manageable and do not mean the medicine is unsafe. Still, keeping track of how your body responds is important. If the mild symptoms become bothersome or do not go away, it's a good idea to bring them up with your healthcare provider for reassurance or advice.

Rare but Serious Risks

While Tylenol 8 Hour is widely trusted and safe when used correctly, it does carry some rare but serious risks. The most important one is liver damage. Taking more than the recommended dose or combining acetaminophen with alcohol can put a heavy strain on the liver. This may lead to serious illness, which can even be life-threatening if ignored. Another rare but serious reaction is an allergic response. Signs of this might include swelling of the face or throat, severe rash, or difficulty breathing. In some very uncommon cases, acetaminophen has been linked to skin reactions that can become dangerous if untreated. People who have existing liver disease, drink alcohol often, or take other medicines that affect the liver should be extra cautious. These risks are rare, but because of their seriousness, it's essential to stick strictly to the dosage instructions and avoid mixing medicines without professional advice. The good news is that when used responsibly, most people never encounter these severe problems, and the benefits outweigh the risks.

When to Seek Medical Attention

Knowing when to call for medical help is one of the most important parts of using Tylenol 8 Hour safely. If you notice severe stomach pain, yellowing of the skin or eyes (a sign of liver trouble), or very dark urine, you should seek help immediately. These may point to liver injury, which needs quick treatment. You should also get urgent medical attention if you develop swelling in your face or throat, severe rash, or trouble breathing, as these may signal an allergic reaction. Even if you are unsure, it's always better to be cautious. If you accidentally take more than the recommended amount, do not wait for symptoms—contact your doctor or emergency services right away. Another sign to look out for is ongoing pain that does not improve even after regular doses. This could mean you need a different type of treatment or that another condition is present. Remember, your body often gives warning signs when something is wrong. Listening to these signals and acting quickly can prevent serious harm. When in doubt, reaching out to a doctor or pharmacist is always the safest choice.

Chapter 5: Maximizing Benefits and Managing Pain

Lifestyle and Complementary Approaches

Living with arthritis pain doesn't always have to rely only on tablets. Simple changes in your lifestyle can make a big difference. Gentle exercise like walking, swimming, or yoga helps keep your joints flexible and reduces stiffness. Moving every day, even for short periods, prevents your muscles from weakening. Another key factor is diet. Eating foods rich in omega-3 fatty acids, like salmon, walnuts, and flaxseeds, can help reduce inflammation. Staying hydrated and maintaining a healthy weight also eases the strain on your joints. Stress is another hidden factor that can worsen pain. Practices like meditation, breathing exercises, or even listening to calm music can relax your body and mind. Some people also find comfort in complementary therapies such as massage, heat therapy, or acupuncture. These do not replace medication but can add extra relief and improve overall well-being. The goal is balance—supporting your body naturally while letting the tablets handle pain control when needed. Over time, these small habits create a foundation for healthier joints and a more active lifestyle.

Combining with Other Treatments Safely

While Tylenol 8 Hour Arthritis Pain Tablets can be effective, many people also use other treatments. It is very important to combine them safely. Acetaminophen can often be taken with non-medication methods like physical therapy, stretching routines, or applying hot and cold packs. These do not interfere with the medicine. However, caution is needed when mixing with other drugs. For example, avoid taking multiple products that also contain acetaminophen, as this increases the risk of liver damage. Some people may be prescribed non-steroidal anti-inflammatory drugs (NSAIDs), like ibuprofen, but these should only be combined if approved by a healthcare provider. Supplements, such as glucosamine or turmeric, are generally considered safe but should still be mentioned to your doctor, as they might interact with other prescriptions. If you use alcohol or herbal remedies, it is important to be upfront about it, because they can affect how your body processes acetaminophen. The best approach is to create a clear treatment plan with your doctor or pharmacist. This way, you can get the benefit of different therapies without increasing risks. Safe combination means more effective and reliable pain control in the long run.

Tips for Long-Term Pain Management

Arthritis pain often requires long-term strategies, not just quick fixes. One of the most important steps is consistency—taking your medicine as directed and not skipping doses. Tracking your pain levels in a journal can help you notice patterns, like weather changes or certain activities that trigger more discomfort. This information is valuable for adjusting your daily routine. Long-term management also includes pacing yourself. Overdoing physical tasks can lead to flare-ups, so learn to balance activity with rest. Sleep is another cornerstone of pain control. A regular bedtime routine, a supportive mattress, and avoiding screens before sleep can improve rest, which in turn reduces pain sensitivity. Building a support system is equally vital. Talking with family, joining arthritis support groups, or speaking to a counselor helps you stay motivated and less isolated. Setting realistic goals, like walking an extra five minutes a day or cooking more anti-inflammatory meals, keeps progress steady without overwhelming you. Remember that arthritis management is not about perfection—it's about small, steady steps that improve your quality of life. With patience, planning, and the right habits, long-term pain can be managed effectively while allowing you to live a fulfilling life.

Conclusion

Key Takeaways for Safe and Effective Relief

When using Tylenol 8 Hour Arthritis Pain Tablets, safety and effectiveness go hand in hand. First, always follow the recommended dosage instructions. Taking more than advised will not relieve pain faster and can seriously harm your liver. Consistency matters too. Taking the tablets at evenly spaced intervals ensures continuous relief throughout the day and prevents pain from returning. Keep track of your total acetaminophen intake if you use other medicines or cold and flu remedies to avoid accidental overdose. Listening to your body is equally important—if pain persists or worsens despite following the instructions, consult your doctor rather than increasing the dose. Store the tablets in a cool, dry place, away from children, to maintain their effectiveness. Avoid alcohol while using acetaminophen, as it increases the risk of liver damage. Lastly, remember that Tylenol provides relief, not a cure. Combining it with gentle exercise, proper rest, and healthy habits can significantly improve your overall comfort and mobility. By keeping these points in mind, you can safely use Tylenol 8 Hour to manage arthritis pain effectively, giving yourself the best chance to stay active and enjoy daily life.

Questions to Ask Your Healthcare Provider

Talking to your healthcare provider is a crucial step when managing arthritis pain. Before starting Tylenol 8 Hour, ask about your personal risk factors. Questions like, "Is this safe for my liver?" or "Could this interact with my other medications?" help prevent complications. If you have chronic conditions, such as kidney or liver issues, make sure to discuss them so your provider can guide your dosage safely. Ask about long-term use and whether there are alternative pain management options if your pain increases over time. Understanding side effects is important too—questions like, "What should I do if I notice unusual symptoms?" or "When should I seek urgent care?" ensure you are prepared for any situation. You can also ask about lifestyle adjustments that may complement the medication, such as exercise routines, dietary choices, or other non-drug therapies. Being proactive with your questions empowers you to make informed decisions about your care, reduces the risk of complications, and helps you manage pain effectively. A thoughtful conversation with your healthcare provider can transform your approach to arthritis management and give you peace of mind.

Final Thoughts on Living Well with Arthritis

Living well with arthritis goes beyond taking pain medicine—it's about embracing a lifestyle that supports mobility, comfort, and overall health. Tylenol 8 Hour can relieve pain, but combining it with daily habits like gentle stretching, low-impact exercises, and maintaining a healthy weight can make a real difference. Pay attention to your body and pace yourself; avoid pushing through severe pain, but don't let mild discomfort stop you from staying active. Diet plays a role too—foods rich in antioxidants, omega-3s, and vitamins can help reduce inflammation naturally. Adequate rest and stress management are equally important, as fatigue and tension can worsen pain. Connecting with support networks, whether friends, family, or arthritis support groups, can provide encouragement and practical advice. Remember, small consistent actions often have a bigger impact than dramatic changes. With careful attention, patience, and a holistic approach, it is possible to live an active, fulfilling life even with arthritis. Using Tylenol 8 Hour as part of this strategy allows you to manage discomfort, maintain independence, and focus on enjoying your daily activities without letting pain define you.

Printed in Dunstable, United Kingdom

71416839R00025